YOU: STRESS LESS

The Owner's Manual for Regaining Balance in Your Life

MICHAEL F. ROIZEN, MD
MEHMET C. OZ, MD

FREE PRESS

New York   London   Toronto   Sydney   New Delhi

DISCLAIMER

This publication contains the opinions and ideas of its authors. It is intended to provide helpful and informative material on the subjects addressed in the publication. It is sold with the understanding that the authors and publisher are not engaged in rendering medical, health, or any other kind of personal professional services in the book. The reader should consult his or her medical, health, or other competent professional before adopting any of the suggestions in this book or drawing inferences from it.

The authors and publisher specifically disclaim all responsibility for any liability, loss, or risk, personal or otherwise, which is incurred as a consequence, directly or indirectly, of the use and application of any of the contents of this book.

FREE PRESS
A Division of Simon & Schuster, Inc.
1230 Avenue of the Americas
New York, NY 10020

First Free Press trade paperback edition October 2011

FREE PRESS and colophon are trademarks of Simon & Schuster, Inc.

For information about special discounts for bulk purchases,
please contact Simon & Schuster Special Sales at 1-866-506-1949
or business@simonandschuster.com.

The Simon & Schuster Speakers Bureau can bring authors to your live event.
For more information or to book an event contact the Simon & Schuster Speakers
Bureau at 1-866-248-3049 or visit our website at www.simonspeakers.com.

Manufactured in the United States of America

1 3 5 7 9 10 8 6 4 2

ISBN 978-1-4516-4074-8
ISBN 978-1-4516-5907-8 (ebook)

To YOU who feel stressed . . .
May you learn to make stress beneficial
and be younger, healthier, and more "beautiful
inside and out."

The You Docs

Stress Less, Live More

In a world where you have more information, more responsibilities, more electronic devices, and more ways to update your status, it's no wonder that you also have more stress.

Why? Because in response to all of the increased demands on you, you search for more, too. You want more time, more money, more energy, more sleep, more IT support, more friends to follow, more reality shows to take your minds off the heavy stuff in your lives.

So what's the result? You may end up on the wrong end of stress's right hook. And it beats you up. Badly.

The truth is, many people actually misunderstand stress. Many believe that the secret to eliminating stress is, well, eliminating stress. While bubble baths and island living may be the answer for some, stress-elimination isn't really the goal. You actually need stress—and many stresses are actually good for your health. The secret, then, is figuring out what's good, what's bad, and then using that information to minimize the destructive effects of certain stresses, so you can lead a healthy and happy life.

In this book, you'll find seventy-five of our best "Stress Less" secrets culled from the research we did for several of our bestselling books in the *YOU: The Owner's Manual* series. Within these pages, you'll find some big-picture lessons that will help you redefine what stress is, and you'll come across dozens of nuggets that will help you in a pinch—to sleep better, feel more energized, and be ready to embrace all of the wonderful things that life has to offer.

Now, if you'll excuse us, we're off to do some meditation . . . "ommmmmmmmmmmmmmmmm."

Here's to a healthy and happy YOU,
Michael F. Roizen, MD, and Mehmet C. Oz, MD

YOU:
STRESS
LESS

STRESS:
THE BIG PICTURE

1. Know the Difference
We tend to think that stress is like a pair of slippers—one size fits all. Either we're stressed, or we're not. But the fact is that stress comes in different shapes, sizes, and levels of intensity. Some of us certainly worry more than others, and some of us are much better equipped to cope with exploding dishwashers than others. But the danger is that stress—which often increases as we age—is a major driver of many kinds of health problems. It's important to know the different kinds of stress you experience. They are:

Ongoing Low-level Stress or Single-event Stress: You work, you have a family, you interact with people who sometimes sneeze without covering their mouths. Life generates a constant hum of stress, no matter who you are or what you do (i.e., your babysitter fails to show up and you have to hustle your kids off to a surprisingly accommodating sister-in-law). To expect that you can eliminate all stress is not only unreasonable but also unhealthy because, as you'll see in a moment, your ability to respond to stress can make you stronger. You deal with it. Stress over.

Nagging Unfinished Tasks: One of the most influential forms of stress comes in the form of a chisel that chips and chips and chips and chips and chips and chips away at your brain cells a little bit at a time. Until. You. Can't. Take. It. *Any freaking more!* Whether it's a cluttered closet, or cracked bathroom tiles that have been staring at you for years, or weekly paperwork that gnaws at you every Friday, these nagging unfinished tasks (we call them NUTs) are much more destructive than the low levels of stress we expect from life.

Major Life Events: You don't need us to tell you the kinds of things that fit this category; a divorce, a move, a job change, a death in the family, a sudden serious illness, and bankruptcy aren't exactly on the same level as a cell-phone battery dying. The stats show that three major life events in a one-year period will make your body feel and act as though it were thirty-two years older in the following year—meaning that it's especially important to develop coping strategies and support systems to sustain you in times of crisis.

2. Remember, Some Stress Can Be Good

Stress is good. There, we said it. Instead of calling us crazier than a four-headed firefly, hear us out. Stress heightens all of our biological systems so we can deal with an impending threat, be it an enemy, a natural disaster, or the fact that some idiot built the fire too close to the cave. Changes occur inside our body that give us the strength or the sense to fight a predator or hightail it out of there. What happens to your body during high-intensity stress? Your concentration becomes more focused than a microscope, your reaction time becomes faster, and your strength increases exponentially. Historically, stress was good—it kept you alive.

3. Until It Backfires

The big difference between stress today and stress yesterday isn't the fact that cavemen didn't have e-mail; it's that their stress was fleeting. They had periods of high-intensity stress (a saber-toothed tiger up ahead!) followed by low (or no) levels (whew, it passed by the cave). Though our cave ancestors did have some big stresses, like famine, it's a bit different today. Today we're drowning in a sea of stress, with wave after wave after wave knocking us over. Those heightened biological reactions work in our favor for short periods, but when stress continues unabated, those biological reactions turn wacky.

4. Understand the Threats, Seize the Opportunity

Simply, too much stress can lead to a host of ultimate stress-enders, like heart attacks, cancer, and disabling accidents. Plus, stress weakens your immune system and destroys your sleep patterns, which can lead to unhealthy addictions to food, alcohol, or 3 a.m. infomercials. And that's not even counting the other things that stress is associated with, like depression, alcohol and tobacco addictions, mood disorders, headaches, and fatigue. You get it: If you can reduce the effects of your stress and increase your effectiveness in stress-management, you'll live a much healthier and happier life.

5. Learn Some Biology

Before we tell you what you can do to manage your stress, we believe it's important to learn how stress works—and why it can be so destructive. When you learn the why, you'll be better equipped to handle the how-to.

Essentially, stress symptoms are experienced when a series of chemicals that are produced in your brain travel through your blood and affect just about every system in your body. Specifically, this happens through the stress circuit—the interaction between your nervous system and your stress hormones. That's the hormonal system that sounds like a *Star Wars* galaxy: the hypothalamic-pituitary-adrenal (HPA) axis.

The stress hormones cycle among these three glands in a feedback loop. When you're faced with a major stressor like a mugger, a looming deadline, or a chocolate shortage, the cone-shaped hypothalamus at the base of your brain releases CRH (corticotrophin-releasing hormone), which then does a hula dance on your pituitary gland, stimulating it to release *another* hormone called ACTH (adrenocorticotropic hormone) into your bloodstream. ACTH signals your adrenal glands to release cortisol and facilitates production and then release of epinephrine (also known as adrenaline, the fight-or-flight chemical). These four chemicals serve as your body's SWAT team—they respond to emergencies. Adrenaline increases your blood pressure and heart rate, while cortisol releases sugar in the form of glucose to fuel your muscles and your mind. Then, to close the loop, cortisol travels back to the hypothalamus to stop the production of CRH. Stress over, hormones released, body returns to normal. But only if the stress stops as well.

6. Learn Some *More* Biology

In addition to giving you the chemical tools to beat the dickens out of your stressors, stress hormones also work throughout various regions of the brain to influence everything from mood and fear to memory and appetite. And they also interact with hormonal systems that control reproduction, metabolism, and immunity. See where this is going? The HPA axis is like a curious two-year-old, touching everything in its path. That's okay in short spurts, but not when you overfill your hormonal systems. That's why stress is so highly correlated with bad health. Specifically, this is what happens when you let the hormones in the HPA axis run crazy:

❑ An overactive HPA axis can mean that your body is unable to turn off your stress response. So? That can lead to anxiety and depression, which are further manifested through such things as low sex drive and high blood pressure. Also it leads to graying of your hair prematurely (perhaps why presidential hair often turns gray in office).

❏ When the HPA axis is flooded, we also experience other potentially fatal health problems, like elevated lousy LDL cholesterol or triglycerides combined with reduced healthy HDL cholesterol, not to mention rupture of vulnerable plaques. Part of this risk comes from a stress-related surge in chemicals called cannabinoids, which cause us to eat and can eventually lead to such conditions as diabetes and the biggie (literally), obesity.

❏ Cortisol prevents the release of chemicals that strengthen your immune system. That's why you tend to get sick when you're stressed out. Too much cortisol essentially suppresses your immune system and decreases your ability to fight infection. Stress also makes you more susceptible to diseases that you rely on your immune system to hold at bay or eradicate, like cancer. Men have a pretty quick rebound from the cortisol release during stress, but women often sense a lingering impact of the hormone, which is why men are so chipper the day after a lover's spat that they have already forgotten about it, while women retain perfect recall of the event, together with the emotional undertones. CRH prevents the release of a hormone that controls all the hormones responsible for reproduction and sexual behavior, including those that control ovulation and sperm release. Indeed, reducing stress is one of the tactics used by couples with fertility issues. They're relaxing not just for some mumbo-jumbo reason but to try to make their bodies better equipped hormonally for conception. Makes evolutionary sense, right? Why would you want to produce babies in the middle of a drought or when fighting off hairy four-legged neighbors?

❑ If the HPA axis is activated for too long, it hinders the release of growth hormone. As you'll learn in future chapters, you need your own (natural) growth hormone to help combat some diseases and conditions and to build lean muscle mass. If you keep the axis activated for too long, it can develop an exhausted response—and that produces a wiped-out feeling when stress does come.

7. Learn Why Stress Can Make You Fat

Chronic stress triggers an ancient response of calorie accumulation and fat storage, so we end up continually upgrading the size of our omentum storage unit (the omentum is the fat-storing organ near your stomach). Here's where the cycle of fat spins out of control:

❑ When you have chronic stress, your body increases its production of steroids and insulin, which . . .

❑ Increases your appetite, which . . .

7

❏ Increases the chance you'll engage in hedonistic eating in the form of high-calorie sweets and fats, which . . .

❏ Makes you store more fat, especially in the omentum, which . . .

❏ Pumps more fat and inflammatory chemicals into the liver, which . . .

❏ Creates a resistance to insulin, which . . .

❏ Makes your pancreas secrete more insulin to compensate, which . . .

❏ Makes you hungrier than a muzzled wolf, which . . .

❏ Continues the cycle of eating, because you're stressed and being stressed because you're eating.

STRESS-MANAGEMENT TECHNIQUES:
HEALTHY LIFESTYLE BASICS

8. Get Eight

Blame it on the invention of electricity, more demanding jobs, or great late-night TV, but we sleep a whole lot less nowadays than we used to. On average, Americans awake at 5:47 a.m. and do not hit the bed (not when we actually sleep) until after 10:15 p.m.; that may not be enough. You need eight hours to feel restored, to have energy, to let your body's systems and chemicals re-charge and thrive. Good sleep will help you manage your energy systems— essential for fighting stress.

9. Keep the Bedroom Sacred

Do nothing in your bedroom but sleep and have sex. If you work, watch TV, or work out to fitness DVDs in the room, you're basically training your body to be alert in the bedroom space. Your bedroom should be a sanctuary from the normal hustle and bustle of life.

10. Practice Good Sleep Hygiene

That means you should make a sleep schedule (plan your eight hours); before that eight-hour period starts, give yourself ten minutes to do the quick chores absolutely needed for the next day (such as making lunch), another ten minutes for hygiene, and ten minutes for meditation (all before starting the eight hours). Some people even dim the lights in their bedroom an hour before sleep to transition from artificial light to darkness. Another helper: Make sure your room is cool; the ideal sleep temp seems to be around 67 degrees.

11. Add in a Power Nap

Just make sure to keep it under thirty minutes. Any longer than that, and you'll slip into a stage of deeper sleep so close to the dreamy REM phase that when awakened from it, you'll feel hung over and drowsy (that feeling, by the way, is called sleep inertia and is associated with making bad financial judgments and getting into auto accidents). At less than thirty minutes, a nap can be invigorating. Naps enable your body and brain to reboot and are commonly practiced in societies that boast great energy and longevity.

12. Get Some Aid

In terms of sleep supplements, the data aren't good enough to love these, but some patients like valerian root (though it has an energizing effect in 10 percent of people), passion flower, theanine, hops (ask any college student), and melatonin (0.5 to 3 mg, especially if you're jet-lagged or working weird shift hours). Calcium (600 mg) and magnesium (300 mg) are also helpful. These can help you get to sleep and wake up refreshed with no hangover (which some sleep drugs cause). Or try an essential oil aromatherapy for sleep (see your local health food store or www.shopascents.com).

13. Use Food in Your Favor

We think food is nature's best medicine, especially when it comes to maintaining energy levels throughout the day. Higher energy levels will most effectively help you manage stress and avoid the ups and downs that can come from eating unhealthy foods. Practicing healthy eating habits (eating a balance of lean protein, healthy carbohydrates, and healthy fats) will help you manage the ups and downs that can come from classic stress eating (doughnut, STAT!). Aim to consume high-quality protein such as nuts and fish and a low-carb diet, and include lots of fruits, vegetables, and 100 percent whole grains.

14. Drink Up

Drink as much water as it takes to keep your mouth and lips moist throughout the day, so that your urine is clear enough to read through. One hidden cause of fatigue is a little bit of dehydration. It's something that many people can't quite identify, so if you're feeling a little low, a glass of water (and not a bag of M&M's) may be the jolt you really need.

15. Avoid Simple Sugars

They end in -ose, like glucose, sucrose, maltose, dextrose, etc. (except ribose!). Also, avoid syrups (another word for sugar), any grain but 100 percent whole grains (since processed grains turn into simple sugars and increase your blood sugar quickly), and saturated and trans fats.

16. Go Turkey
Turkey contains tryptophan, which increases serotonin to improve your mood, combat depression, and help you resist cravings for simple carbs. But turkey isn't the greatest source of tryptophan. Try chicken soup and dark chocolate (preferably not in the same bowl).

17. Develop a List of Emergency Foods
They can satisfy you when cravings get the best of you—things like V8 juice, a handful of nuts, fruit, cut-up vegetables, or even a little guacamole.

18. Change the Temptation
Eating out at a colorful fast-food joint is like rowing out to a hurricane. The savory foods will flip you like a tidal wave. So the first trick to eating out is choosing a place that offers many healthy options (or will make them for you). You should be especially aware of danger zones such as the first ten minutes of the meal (order veggies and olive oil, instead of bread) and the last ten minutes (have your glass of wine at the end of the meal, rather than a slab of chocolate mousse cake).

19. Manage the Drive-Through
We understand how it is. Sometimes you need the absolute quickest path from food to belly, especially when you're

moving quickly between a lot of different responsibilities. While most fast-food options are more destructive than a 4 a.m. vandal, you can still make smart choices in the drive-through lane. Some things to remember:

- ❑ There are some main dishes that can be good for you, but you have to be careful. Some slight name variations can make the difference between causing your fat and keeping you flat.
- ❑ Avoid side dishes and desserts. They're mostly loaded with bad fats and simple sugars, and they often have more calories than the main dishes.
- ❑ Choose low-calorie dressing, not low-fat. Low-fat dressings are steeped in HFCS, which has plenty of calories, and the fructose tricks your body into staying hungry.

20. Make This for Breakfast

Pineapple-Banana Protein Blaster
2 servings; 207 calories per serving

1 large ripe banana, broken into chunks
½ cup low-fat (1 percent) soy milk
1 can (4 ounces) crushed pineapple in juice, undrained
½ cup pineapple-passion fruit sorbet
1 tablespoon soy protein powder (8 grams protein)

Combine all ingredients in blender. Cover; blend until fairly smooth.

21. Make This to Have on Hand

Garden Harvest Soup

10 servings (about 1 cup each); 176 calories per serving

1 tablespoon extra-virgin olive oil

1 medium onion, chopped

1 carrot, chopped

4 garlic cloves, thinly sliced

1 red bell pepper, chopped

2 quarts (8 cups) low-salt vegetable or chicken stock or broth

1 can (28 ounces) whole, crushed, or diced tomatoes, undrained

2 cups water

1 small head cabbage, thinly sliced

½ teaspoon hot red pepper sauce (optional)

Salt and freshly ground black pepper (optional)

Optional garnishes: chopped fresh parsley, chopped fresh cilantro

Heat a large saucepan over medium-high heat. Add oil, then onion; cook 5 minutes, stirring occasionally. Stir in carrot, garlic, and bell pepper; cook until tender. Add stock, tomatoes, water, and cabbage; simmer uncovered 20 minutes. Season to taste with hot sauce and salt and pepper if desired. Garnish with parsley or cilantro if desired.

22. Turn Bad Food Good

Stuffed Whole Wheat Pizza

4 servings (2 slices per serving); for the first two weeks,
you can have up to half of the pizza, but most will not need
that much to be full • 322 calories per serving

Cooking oil spray

1 pound fresh stir-fry vegetables such as asparagus, broccoli,
   cauliflower, mushrooms, multicolored bell peppers, red
   and white onions, and zucchini, cut up

2 garlic cloves, minced

Salt and freshly ground black pepper (optional)

1 cup pizza sauce or tomato sauce

2 tablespoons olive relish or tapenade

2 tablespoons sundried-tomato bits

One 12-inch or 10-ounce prepared thin whole wheat pizza crust

1/2 cup (2 ounces) finely shredded part-skim mozzarella cheese

Heat oven to 425°F. Heat a large nonstick skillet over medium-high.
Heat until hot; coat with cooking spray. Add vegetables and garlic; stir-fry
(really sauté) 2 to 5 minutes, or until vegetables are crisp-tender. Season to
taste with salt and pepper if desired. Combine pizza sauce, olive relish, and
sundried-tomato bits. Spread over pizza crust; top with cooked vegetables
and cheese. Bake pizza directly on oven rack 10 to 15 minutes, or until crust
is golden brown and cheese is melted. Cut pizza into 8 wedges.

23. Choose the Energy Vitamin

You need B vitamins for your mitochondria (your body's power plants) to produce energy from glucose. Most of us absorb the B vitamins well (in either liquid or pill form), but 99 percent of us don't get enough from our diets. Take half a multivitamin (pill splitters cost less than two dollars) in the morning and evening (twice a day to keep stable levels, since we pee the water-soluble vitamins out) to keep you energized. You may want to get your vitamin B12 and D3 levels checked yearly. You may be the rare person who doesn't absorb them well from your stomach and intestine and needs a B12 vitamin injection yearly, or 3000 IU daily (in pill form) of vitamin D3.

24. Go Green

Green tea has been shown to have a very high content of polyphenols, which are chemicals with potent antioxidant properties (believed to be greater than even vitamin C's). They give tea its bitter flavor. Because green tea leaves are young and have not been oxidized, green tea has up to 40 percent polyphenols, while black tea contains only about 10 percent. Green tea has one-third the caffeine of black tea, but it's been shown to yield the same level of energy and attentiveness in more even levels than the ups and downs associated with other caffeinated drinks. Just don't drink milk with it; the casein in milk has been shown to inhibit the beneficial effects of tea.

25. If You Choose an Energy Drink, Choose Carefully

"Energy" drinks seem to have taken over the world—you can get them everywhere from convenience stores to nightclubs. But the question is, do they work? We wish we could give a definitive answer, but there are just not enough data to be sure. If you are going to indulge, go for the ones with the lowest sugar content. Many are loaded with caffeine or its equivalent, which, of course, can explain why drinkers feel a boost, no matter what the other "energy" ingredients are (things like taurine and guarana).

26. Embrace Chia

Say the word *chia*, and most of us immediately think of little green pets. But we want you to think of chia for another reason: A whole grain used by the Aztecs as their main energy source, chia can help restore energy levels and decrease inflammation because of its omega-3 fatty acids. Similar to cornstarch, chia can be used as a thickening agent and as a substitute for whole grains in your diet. Whole grains, of course, are especially important because they help stabilize blood sugar levels, as opposed to causing the spikes and falls that can occur when you eat sugars and refined carbohydrates, which contribute to fluctuating energy levels.

27. Sock It Up

Sometimes, after a hard day, your legs may feel as though they have about as much zip as if you were a napping cat. They feel heavy, you feel tired, and the only thing you want your legs to do is hang out on the ottoman. One solution: socks or stockings that compress your feet, calves, and thighs. Besides giving you the benefit of decreasing the chance of developing varicose veins, these stockings—after a day of wear—will make your legs feel stronger and better rested. How? They decrease the pooling of blood in your legs, letting your heart function better. Though the best stockings are custom-made, off-the-shelf ones work well, too; choose ones with pressures starting at 10 mmHg and work up to 40 mmHg. The higher the pressure, the better they work, but the more expensive they will be and the harder they are to put on. You can wear compression stockings every day for about four months (that's when they usually wear out), washing them in cold water at night.

28. Get Rid of Infections

While most of us want to treat infections because of their acute symptoms, we can't ignore that they can have chronic implications as well. Since inflammation and infection can be two of the dominos in the cascade of low-energy symptoms, one of your goals should be to monitor your body so that infections don't linger. That means regular flossing to decrease the risk of gum inflammation, regular use of a neti pot to reduce sinusitis, and probiotics for treating such infections as prostatitis, bowel infections, and vaginitis. Many infections are viral, in which case good sleep, frequent hand washing, and food choices that avoid all simple sugars and saturated fats can help.

29. Be a Marine

And stand up straight, would ya? Good posture promotes strong core muscles—and helps you feel energized all day. Bad posture? Well, let's just say it teaches your muscles to crumble like a cookie. Correct posture should be practiced with your back against a wall. Tucking your chin under slightly will allow a larger area of the back of your head to touch the wall, as well as the top of your back, buttocks, and legs. The small of the back should not be against the wall (the spine is naturally curved). Pretend a string attached to the top of your skull is pulling you skyward, and feel yourself becoming taller. When you're standing for a long time, elevate one foot on a step or curb to help alleviate some pressure. And if you're sitting for a long time, put your feet up on a stool, so your knees are higher than your hips; that will decrease the pressure on the discs in your lower back.

30. Watch *The Daily Show*

When we laugh, natural killer cells that destroy tumors and viruses increase, but there's more. Laughing lowers blood pressure, increases oxygen in the blood with deeper respirations, and helps address the effect of mental stress on the arteries. And you can't beat the price.

31. But Go Ahead and Cry

Boys and girls cry an equal amount until age thirteen, and then guys cut down to once a month while gals stay at once a week. Women must realize that tears lubricate the soul.

According to the research, crying may serve as a request for help or to communicate the presence of a problem such as hunger, pain, or loneliness, and it may serve as a signal of empathy. Tears flow in response to watching a fellow human being in trouble, as well as through some sort of de-stressing mechanism after arousal. Technically, the parasympathetic nervous system is what shoots out tears via nerve messages. The program is especially active when people experience moods and emotions characterized by helplessness—which explains why we cry when we're sad or hurt or stressed. The actual content of tears, in case you're wondering, is a chemical cocktail of various hormones such as estrogen, prolactin (the same stuff that helps women breast-feed offspring), and proteins. What's even more amazing is that the substance of tears actually differs depending on whether the tears are generated by emotions or simply for the purpose of lubricating dry eyes.

32. Identify Your Mood

Recent research shows what many of us knew all along: Our moods dictate what we eat. Researchers studied the diets of people to show how personality and foods collide— how our moods may steer us to certain foods on the basis of their physical characteristics. The study theorized that many moods send specific signals; for example, stressed adrenal glands could be sending salt-craving signals. So what does your favorite turn-to food say about you? Tough foods, like meat, or hard and crunchy foods: angry.

Sugars: depressed. Soft and sweet foods, like ice cream: anxious. Salty foods: stressed. Bulky, fill-you-up foods, like crackers and pasta: lonely and/or sexually frustrated. Anything and everything: jealous.

33. Play

It is important to integrate some playtime into the busiest of schedules. Laughing, playing, and relaxing all decrease your stress level. Play actually decreases your levels of the stress hormones cortisol and adrenaline, while distracting you from the source of the stress. Daydreaming can have a similar effect: Imagine yourself on a great vacation with your best friend and all the freedom in the world. It could be on a beach, at your favorite place in a city, or somewhere exotic and unknown. Sound like paradise? It turns out it's more than that; that quick mental image actually improves your brain function, keeping your brain flexible and getting those creative juices flowing.

34. Hang Out

Friends are the ultimate de-stressor. Research shows that one of the most vital elements in reducing the negative health effects of stress is to have strong social networks. It's mental medicine. And evidence shows that interacting with a good friend actually lowers your blood pressure and makes you more productive. However, there can be too much of a good thing, especially in today's social-network-driven world. A virtual social life, including pressure to constantly check the latest updates on Facebook, or to tweet or text back in response to each IM, can be a stressor in and of itself. Carving out face time with your friends rather than a constant barrage of Facebook posts may be a better de-stressor. In women, it has been shown that high stress levels stimulate a surge of the bonding hormone oxytocin in the brain, causing women to want to get together and have coffee—no, really, the drive is for them to get together, talk, and de-stress. When men are stressed, they don't get the same surge of oxytocin, so there is less drive to get together and talk. Sorry, guys, you may have to cultivate other strategies to de-stress if your brain isn't giving you that prod to go hang out. And guys, too, remember friends—they take the stress out of stress management.

STRESS-MANAGEMENT TECHNIQUES:
ACTIVITY

35. Get Moving
Any type of exercise or activity will help reduce stress. Your body will love the endorphins, and you'll experience more energy and lower stress levels if you make activity a regular part of your life. If you're just starting, we recommend walking thirty minutes a day, every day. As you build up, you can integrate other activities, like resistance exercises or other cardiovascular exercises such as swimming or cycling.

36. Invest in This
A great pedometer is one of the four things we think you should overpay for—keeping track of your steps or distance walked helps keep you motivated to move throughout the day (the other things, in case you're wondering, are a heart-rate monitor, a pair of cross-training shoes, and an eight-inch chef's knife).

37. Embrace the Benefits of Yoga
You don't have to be a human rubber band to appreciate the beauty of yoga. This ancient practice not only stretches

your muscles but also allows your mind to focus and trains your brain for meditation. The beauty of this workout is that any skill level can participate; you need to move only as far into each pose as you possibly can. In fact, the only imperative you have to remember is to take deep belly breaths using your diaphragm to pull your lungs down during inspiration. (If the poses we outline below are too difficult for you to take continuous deep breaths, then back off to avoid compromising this golden rule.) That's important because most of us never take a single deep breath all day long. It is important—deep breathing stimulates your vagus nerve, and that quiets and calms your brain and stress response. Or as we say— what happens to vagus doesn't stay there, it relaxes your brain. To exhale, suck your belly button toward your spine to push the diaphragm up and empty all the air from your lungs. Inhaling deeply brings a chemical called nitric oxide from the back of your nose and your sinuses into your lungs. This short-lived gas dilates the air passages in your lungs and the blood vessels surrounding those air passages so you can get more oxygen into your body. Nitric oxide also doubles as a neurotransmitter to help your brain function. Other benefits of yoga:

❑ Yoga trains you to loosen the muscles and joints that
   are ignored in your day-to-day life. Routines get the
   blood flowing as you warm up and free your body
   to experience the new stresses you will inevitably
   face each day. The practice also helps you handle the

weight of your body more effectively, which builds bone and muscle strength so you are more resilient. And it improves your balance so you don't fall.

❑ Yoga also helps you to focus your mind on remote parts of your body, such as tight joints and muscles, as you gently but firmly deepen into your poses. Attaining the "empty" mind called for in meditation proves difficult, especially for novices, but if you can concentrate on the tension in your hip, for example, then you're well on your way. The goal in yoga is not really emptying your mind, but rather freeing the mind to let any and all ideas rapidly pass through it without any attachment.

38. Follow the Yoga Guidelines

Yoga is designed to help you feel empowered and build your self-discipline. Follow these guidelines to improve your yoga experience:

❑ Never force a pose so you feel a painful strain. Go to where it feels comfortable.

❑ If your knees feel discomfort, use a rolled-up towel, pillow, or blanket as a cushion behind the knee joints.

❑ Resist locking your elbows.

❑ If a pose is difficult to balance, stand against the wall. Your balance may be different from one day to the next. Imbalance during poses may mean an imbalance in other parts of life.

39. to 42. Do These to Loosen Up

1. *Standing Twist*
Warms up spine; loosens body

With your feet shoulder-width apart (mountain pose) and your knees slightly bent with relaxed arms, twist your upper body loosely from side to side. Look where you are going. Breathe normally for thirty seconds.

2. *Standing Leaning Stretch*
Opens lower back and obliques

Interweave your hands and turn them palm side up above your head. Take a deep inhale, and exhale as you stretch to the right; inhale and come back to center, and exhale to the left. Do five times.

3. *X*
Warms up upper body

With your feet in the mountain pose, bring your straight arms up toward the ceiling in a V-shape with the palms facing each other. Inhale and, on the exhale, cross your hands in front of your face, bringing your hands to shoulder height with the palms facing you. Inhale; then exhale and cross your arms again, switching the arm closest to you. The exhale should be sharp and come from your navel. Do continuously for ninety seconds, alternating your arms.

4. *Ladybug*

Opens upper back, neck, and lungs

Inhale deeply and place your fingertips on your shoulders with your elbows out to your sides in line with your shoulders. Keeping your fingers on your shoulders, on the exhale, bring your elbows out in front; keep exhaling and drop your head, bend forward at the neck, and look down to your toes. On the inhale, come back to elbows out to side. Repeat five times.

43. to 47. Do These to Loosen Your Back

1. *Triangle*

Opens spine; helps balance the body

Stand with your right foot pointing directly to the right and your left foot forward at a slight angle. Inhale deeply. As you exhale, move your right hand down your leg toward your right ankle, stopping wherever you feel comfortable, and simultaneously lift your left hand above your head with the palm facing forward. Look up at your left hand, keeping your shoulder parallel to your hip the entire time. Resist trying to twist your shoulders. Take five deep breaths and switch sides. Do twice.

2. *Cat Back/Cow*

Improves flexibility of spine and torso circulation

Get on all fours with your weight evenly distributed; keep your knees under your hips and your wrists under your shoulders. Arms are straight but not locked, and your fingers are spread and facing forward. Start with a straight line from the top of your head to your tailbone. Exhale as you lift your upper back and tuck your tailbone underneath and look toward your belly button, tucking your chin in. Inhale as you reverse into cow and lift your tailbone up; your belly button goes toward the ground. Look straight ahead as the top of your head faces the ceiling. Use your entire spine throughout the movement. Do five times.

3. Extended Cat Stretch
Warms up and awakens entire body; great for your spine

Adding to Cat Back, lift your left knee off the ground and bring it toward your forehead while simultaneously tucking your forehead under. Then inhale and smoothly extend your right leg behind you with pointed toes. Lift your head and look forward. During the entire movement, keep your hips in line and your pelvis steady as you elongate your entire body. Do five times and then switch sides.

4. Thread the Needle
Opens upper back and shoulders

Start on all fours; take your right hand, palm side down, and slide it under your left armpit. Keep extending it as you exhale, and slowly lower your right ear and shoulder to the mat. Simultaneously drop your left elbow onto the mat or as low as feels comfortable. Hold for thirty seconds and switch sides.

5. *Cobra*

Develops strength and flexibility in your back

Lie on your stomach with your hands palm side down under your shoulders, keeping your fingertips directly underneath the tops of your shoulders. Your legs are together and tight like a rock. Point your toes and put your elbows flush against your sides. While looking up at the ceiling, use your spine strength and lift your torso off the floor just to the navel. Resist pressing with your hands and arch your back as much as feels comfortable. Keep your shoulders relaxed and down away from your ears. Hold for twenty seconds.

48. Do This to Lighten Your Legs

Down Dog

Strengthens and stretches the legs and shoulders; energizes the whole body

Start on all fours with your hands shoulder-width apart and your feet hip-width apart. Tuck your toes under. While inhaling, lift your knees off the ground and straighten your legs. Lift your hips back and up and spread your fingers out, pressing your palms flat to the floor. Keep your neck relaxed; your head should be in a neutral position. Lift your quadriceps muscles; keep them activated. Draw your heels toward the floor. Hold for thirty seconds and release back down to the mat while exhaling.

49. Do This to Chill

Corpse
Relaxes entire body

While on your back, let your arms relax down to your sides, palms facing up, extend your legs out straight, and let your feet flop down. With your eyes closed, travel mentally throughout your entire body, relaxing from your toes to the crown of your head. Cover your eyes with a cloth if you like. When you are ready to come up, roll onto your side, hold for fifteen seconds, and then slowly come onto all fours before standing up. Remember to breathe.

STRESS-MANAGEMENT TECHNIQUES:
RELATIONSHIPS

50. Do the Little Things

Sometimes we think that relationships are made or broken on the grand gestures, the big fights, the four-foot teddy bears won at the carnival. But we could strengthen our relationships—and reduce our at-home stress—immensely with more attention to the details (which can help keep the big problems from surfacing). Do something positive every day to "deposit" a good feeling in your relationship—a note on a napkin, a kiss on the cheek, a helping hand on a home project. (If you feel good about yourself, that's also a great gift to give to someone you love.)

51. Make a Date

These days, it's harder and harder to carve out so-called sweetheart time. Plan time together for just the two of you. Share meals when possible, take a walk, hold hands, or just sit on the couch and catch up while the kids are in the other room playing Wii.

52. Compliment Daily

You're never too busy to give compliments. A well-timed "Great hair, honey" can prevent you and your partner from taking each other for granted.

53. Reflect

Remember what your spouse or partner was like when the two of you first started dating. Focus on the characteristics that first attracted you to each other (don't just look there, bucko).

54. Fight Fair

We live in a world that gives us feedback. Our bodies give us feedback when we eat something we don't like (burps). Our computers give us feedback when we boot up. Our stereo speakers give us feedback if we point the mike in the wrong direction (the piercing sound that makes it feel as if blood is coming from your ears!). Funny thing, though: A lot of us have trouble giving feedback to each other—really good, genuine feedback—especially in our romantic relationships. The trouble, of course, is that relationship problems can be an enormous source of stress. Our "feedback" comes off as criticism, snarky remarks, and attacks on character. Use these strategies when you're trying to help each other—to really help, and not hurt, him or her. These are really great to keep in mind when a fight/argument/disagreement is a-brewing.

When giving feedback:

❑ **Be specific:** Feedback must be based on observable behavior, not one's feelings or the conclusions drawn from the behavior. For example, "Thanks for helping the kids build a Lego volcano." Specific compliments help.

❑ **Be timely:** Do it now. Don't let criticisms fester.

❑ **Be actionable:** Make sure it's based on something over which a person has control. "The color of your eyes scares me!" isn't helpful.

❑ **Be positive:** Give both positive and critical feedback, but tip the balance in the positive direction.

When receiving feedback:

❑ Listen without comment, looking directly at the person. When he or she has finished, don't make any statements, but do ask questions if you want clarification. Don't accept, don't deny, and don't rationalize. Because we are rarely taught to give feedback well, you will often get feedback when the giver is angry about something in the moment. Listening should be as active a pursuit as speaking.

❑ Recognize the courage it took to give you the feedback, and consider it a sincere gift intended to help you grow. Thank the giver for the feedback. Make it short but something you can say sincerely, such as "You've really given me something to think about, thanks." It's hard to feel real appreciation when you hear negative messages about your appearance or behavior, so it's important to have simple words of gratitude prepared ahead of time.

❑ Know that feedback can be tough to receive, even if we solicit it and are grateful for it. Although it's simply another's perception, feedback can shake up your feelings about yourself. Plan to do something nice for yourself when you know you're facing tough feedback. Try to do something that bolsters self-esteem—have dinner with friends or engage in an activity that you are particularly good at.

55. Have More Sex

Sex can serve as that nirvana moment between couples—a time when you feel complete happiness and intimacy, a time when you express your love to your mate. In other words, sex is designed to make you feel good. Really, really good. And you don't need us to tell you that those feel-good moments are wonderful ways to help stress melt away. Consider these facts: Men who have sex three times a week can decrease their risk of heart attack and stroke by 50 percent. And women who enjoy sex tend to live longer than those who don't. Great sex makes your body feel and be the equivalent of two to eight years younger.

56. Give Your Spouse Space

A lot of us think that marriage and commitment have to come with a 24/7 contract—you're together all the time.

You live together, you eat together, you vacation together. Heck, you can't even use the bathroom without knowing where your better half is. But partners in any relationship need a little space and can actually thrive on it. They need to live their own lives, as well as develop their own interests and friends. It's unrealistic to expect another person to fulfill your every need. The truth is, couples grow when individuals can remain individuals. Why? Because each of you will bring more back to the marriage if you're relaxed and refreshed.

57. Go Crazy

There's a reason why bungee jumping, river rafting, and sneaking into the supply closet can make the perfect first date. Doing novel things with another person stimulates dopamine—the feel-good chemical that's elevated when you're in love. Also, since men are aroused by fear and anxiety, and heart rates are elevated during both attraction and danger, it increases the likelihood that a man will find his partner more attractive during a daredevil date. The dopamine is actually firing high when you first get together but not necessarily on the eightieth date, so it's even better to make special new adventures or variations more common the longer you're together. Novel choices are especially great for couples whose libido has diminished or whose sex life has gone stale. Stepping out of your norms will help you feel energized in your relationship and in life.

58. Give (and Then Perhaps Receive) a Foot Massage

A good foot rub works for body and mind because:

❑ It elevates levels of oxytocin, which are the hormones that make you feel warm and fuzzy (it's the same hormone that a mother's brain secretes when she's breast-feeding).

❑ It causes arousal, as the foot contains its own set of sexual nerves.

❑ It stimulates lymphatic drainage. Massage helps drain waste material out of your system.

How to do it:

1. Clean up. To make your partner comfortable, clean his or her feet with a warm washcloth or in a shallow basin of warm water.

2. Use the right lotion—one scented with lavender, which is perceived as an aphrodisiac by both men and women. Or just share some lavender aroma.

3. Do the whole foot. In reflexology (which shares some philosophical roots with acupuncture), the foot is seen as a metaphor for the body. The big toe is seen as the top of the head, and the sensitive area at the base of the toes represents the neck. The inner sole of the foot is the belly, while the outer sole is the spine. If an area is bothering your partner, spend some time there to get the good vibes flowing.

4. Work your way up. We store a lot of tension in

our ankles, so move the foot around passively to help relax the joint. Start with the heel and push up toward the leg; pull it down and work it side to side. On the bottoms of the feet, use firm pressure with your thumbs (too light and it'll be ticklish). Use slow, deep pressure, and work the whole foot and in between toes. Pull each toe for ten seconds. Rub the calves from ankle toward knee. Since the calves and feet are farthest from the heart and fighting gravity, it is challenging for them to move lymphatic waste along.

STRESS-MANAGEMENT TECHNIQUES:

MANAGE PAIN

59. Squash a Headache

You know how your belly feels after Thanksgiving dinner when your belt is too tight? A tension headache is the same feeling, but in your head. With nine out of ten women and seven out of ten men experiencing a tension headache sometime during their lives, it's clearly one of the most common pains around. The good news is that it's usually not there all the time and is usually mild or moderate, not drop-to-the-ground severe, like migraine pain. It used to be thought that tension headaches came from muscle tension, but it's now believed that these headaches occur when fluctuations in serotonin and endorphins activate pain pathways in the brain. Tension headaches have more triggers than a rifle range: stress, lack of sleep, skipping meals, bad posture, clenching your teeth, medications, and being about as active as a comatose slug. Your role if you're susceptible to a lot of headaches? Try to find patterns in behavior for when headaches come, then isolate the triggers to see if you can identify the cause and avoid it.

60. Get Touched

Developed in Asia more than two thousand years ago, acupressure works when your fingers press points on the body that release muscular stress. Get a shiatsu massage .

61. . . . or Do It Yourself

You can try these pressure points yourself to relieve tension (lots of experts warn against using these points if you're pregnant):

Belly of your temporalis muscle: Located in the center
of your temple region. Palpate this region with your
first and middle fingers pressed closely together
until you find a tender, muscular zone. If you have
trouble locating this point, place your fingers against
your temples and then clench down on your molars
a few times. You should feel the main belly of your
temporalis muscles bulge in and out.

Behind the ears: Locate the points at the base of the skull
in the back of the head, just behind the bones in back
of the ears, and apply rotational pressure for two
minutes with your thumbs.

Between the eyes: Pinch the tissue just above the nose
with your middle finger near one eye and the thumb
near the other and slowly push upward so you feel
the pressure near your eyebrows.

The hand web: Using the thumb and index finger of the
other hand, apply a pinching pressure to the soft

fleshy web between the thumb and index finger, on the back of the hand.

62. Or Roll on It

Use your spare tennis balls for something other than Bluto's game of fetch. Put one or two balls in a sock. Put the sock under a painful spot in your back and lie on the balls. It works like an ultrafocused deep-tissue massage to relieve tension in the area, sans the hands of Sven.

63. Stop Jawing Around

Nearly 10 percent of the population suffers from pain in the temporomandibular joint (TMJ, so the disease is called TMD). The TMJ is the joint between the upper jaw (called the maxilla) and the lower one (mandible) that purposely dislocates itself with every bite to increase your chewing force. The TMJ is like a hurried business executive—it's constantly on the move. It moves when you're eating, moves when you're talking, moves when you're kissing the neck of your beloved. The edges of these jawbones are coated with slippery connective tissue that allows the bones to move, almost like a silicone pad on a chair leg. If you have some pain in your jaw, you can actually diagnose the problem yourself (untreated, it can lead to headaches, tooth and gum disease, and other problems). Open your jaw. If you feel pain, hear a pop, or can't open your mouth fully, that means you've got some kind of joint problem (causes can be muscular, joint dysfunction, teeth clenching, poor alignment of the teeth, and stress). You should see a TMJ specialist. Besides medication, mouth guards and massage are effective treatments. And more recently, even Botox has been injected into the muscle that clenches the jaw to help relieve the pain.

64. Strengthen Your Neck

Headache pain—a true energy-zapper—can come from weakness or spasms of the neck muscles. You feel the pain in your upper back and it goes to your lower neck, then upper neck, as progressively weak muscles compensate for too much computer or bridge time. If the muscles of your upper back are sore, it may be weakness of the trapezius muscle. Getting symptomatic relief and taking analgesics so you can exercise is the first order of business. Strengthening that area takes five minutes three times a week for ten weeks to reduce such pain by more than 80 percent. See *YOU: Being Beautiful* for a workout that will help strengthen the area.

STRESS-MANAGEMENT TECHNIQUES:
THE SOFTER SIDE

65. Talk It Out

We're living in a world where there's too much talk—we've got talk shows, talking heads, and people who talk the talk but can't walk the walk. Funny, though, in a hyper-communicative society, many of us can't talk about anything other than sports, soaps, or why the media spends so much attention on (fill in celebrity scandal of the day). The fact is, when it comes to reducing the effects of stress and depression, the biggest cure may not be in a pill bottle, but in making sure you don't stay bottled up yourself. Talk therapy probably works through the release of feel-good chemicals, including the bonding hormone oxytocin. Even just talking about your problems with your spouse, friends, or a taxi driver can help. Since women tend to speak much more than men, they may get a much larger brain chemical boost from hashing things out.

66. Use Guided Imagery

Guided imagery isn't the screen of your car's GPS; it's actually a way of making you feel better. The technique has been shown to improve the ability to cope with depression, improve mood, and decrease stress. How do you do it? Go to a quiet place (the bathroom often works well, since privacy is usually respected there). Start by relaxing and breathing deeply (your belly button should move out when you breathe in, and go toward your spine when you exhale), then visualize yourself in different scenarios. Some variations include visualizing yourself in a pleasant place (the beach), fighting disease (seeing your good immune cells fighting off bad germs), or practicing for a big performance (doing well in your job). An example of how guided imagery can cure aches and pains: If you're in pain, visualize the spot of pain. Follow the nerve from that spot to the center of your mind. Ask your body if you can take control of that pain, and visualize the way that would happen.

67. Think about Your Purpose

There are some chemical and biological foundations for the feeling of soul-level satisfaction that comes with finding your own special "it." One theory is that oxytocin, a hormone that is elevated in women after childbirth, also makes you feel a sense of community and pleasure within your family, during a religious experience, or when you have an epiphany about your existence. When levels of oxytocin increase, you feel calm. Another hypothesis argues that your sense of self-esteem and well-being is influenced by the chemical nitric oxide (not to be confused with the laughing gas nitrous oxide). Traits such as hopefulness and optimism are associated with the release of nitric oxide through the body. In the same way, the release of nitric oxide may serve to help reduce feelings of anxiety and stress. But this chemical effect lasts for only seconds, so you need to continually stimulate your body with the right cerebral karma. Whether it's the result of oxytocin, nitric oxide, or both, soul-level satisfaction exists at a biochemical level as well as in your perceptible life. It's your deeper drive—not the drive to fill the needs of your stomach or your muscles or even your mind, but the drive to fill the needs of your soul. So we encourage you to really take some time to think about what drives you and what your passions are. The more you can align your daily activities with them, the calmer and more satisfied you'll feel.

STRESS-MANAGEMENT TECHNIQUES:
IN THE HEAT OF THE MOMENT

68. Create Your Backup Plan

As we said, stress isn't all bad. It's what gives you the concentration and ability to finish a project or meet a deadline. But stress can linger around like week-old leftovers and create its own kind of stink. So in periods of high stress, you need to have a plan that works for you. Such things as exercise and meditation work for some people, and both of them will help you manage chronic stress through the release of such feel-good substances as nitric oxide and brain chemicals called endorphins. But in the heat of the moment, at peak periods of high intensity, you should be able to pull a quick stress-busting behavior out of your biological bag of tricks. Our suggestions:

❑ Scrunch your face tightly for fifteen seconds, then release. Repeat several times. This repetitive contraction and relaxation helps release tension you're holding above the neck.

❑ Breathe in, lick your lips, then blow out slowly. The cool air helps you refocus and slow down.

❑ Cork it. Hold a wine cork vertically between your

teeth. Putting a gentle bite on the cork forces your jaws—a major holder of tension—to relax. (Don't fight stress by emptying the bottle of wine into your body first.)

69. Manage Your Anger

It's no secret that anger doesn't help anyone. Not the fellow motorist you're swearing at. Not the intern you're making cry. Not your kids, who are seeing you lose it. And most of all, not you. Anger has been shown to lead to a higher incidence of heart disease and other health problems. Part of the problem is that we're misinformed about the best way to handle our anger. (By the way, there's a difference between anger, which is frustration at a poor driver, and hostility, which is hoping he runs into the concrete divider.) While you may think that lashing out or hitting a pillow or punching bag helps you release tension, the opposite is true. It teaches you to develop a behavior pattern: Get mad, punch. Get mad, get even. Get mad, harbor stress until it eats away at you like ants on crumbs. Instead, use behavior and mental techniques that have been shown to reduce anger and anxiety, as well as the chronic heart problems associated with them. If you're one of the sixteen million Americans who have anger issues, try these techniques to make a change that we'll all be thankful for:

Do the Opposite: Research has found that "letting it rip" with anger actually escalates anger and aggression and does nothing to help you (or the person you're angry with) resolve the situation. In general, to cope with an emotion, you have to do the opposite. The opposite of anger isn't to withdraw or lash out, but to develop empathy. So instead of swearing at the guy who cut you off, think that maybe there's a reason he did so—like, he just got a call that his wife is in labor or his mom tripped over his child's toy and can't get up. It helps to remind yourself that few people are jerks on purpose. Getting angry just forces you to justify your actions, so you act out to make sense of how crazily you just acted.

Find your pattern: Keep thought records with no censorship of all the emotions you feel (and why) during the day. This helps you identify and find a pattern in the core beliefs that are associated with your anger. Do you get angry at a lack of respect, or wasted time, or insults?

Do push-ups: Somehow you do have to acknowledge that you are experiencing a physiological response to your anger. Telling yourself to "stay calm" is one of the worst things you can do (second only to being told to "calm down"), because we're *supposed* to act out when we feel threatened and are angry. So act out in a way that doesn't burn bridges, by doing push-ups or stretching or deep breathing. This dissipates the physiological burden of anger.

Choose smart words: Be careful of words like *never* or *always* when talking about yourself or someone else.

Expressions such as "This machine never works!" or "You're always forgetting things!" are not only inaccurate, they serve to make you feel that your anger is justified and that there's no way to solve the problem. They also alienate and humiliate people who might otherwise be willing to work with you on a solution. Another important distinction is making sure that you have realistic expectations—and are not blaming yourself for things that aren't under your control, with a string of woulds, coulds, and shoulds.

STRESS-MANAGEMENT TECHNIQUES:
AT WORK

70. Ask If You're in the Right Place

Why do you do what you do? Is it because you love it? Or because you've been successful and make a good salary and, well, it would be a darn shame to give it all up to write Irish poetry for a living? That's essentially the difference between intrinsic motivators (doing something for love, genuine interest, and satisfaction), and external motivators (doing something because some outside influence such as salary motivates you).

In general, intrinsic factors are more important and more stable—and they will help you not only in job situations but also in things such as quitting smoking (better to quit when you're ready, not because somebody nags you to do so). Intrinsic motivations are also self-reinforcing because of our built-in desire to attribute causes to our actions. If we perform a task for an extrinsic reward, we reason that we did the task because of the reward, and not because of something inherently interesting or important in it. But if we perform the task without an extrinsic reward, then we reason that the task itself must be inherently enjoyable or important for us to continue to engage in it. If you work hard on a project for a particular boss, and then the boss moves on (or your feelings about that boss change), you will not keep working hard. But if you work hard because you enjoy the job, this motivation becomes self-reinforcing. You stay engaged in the work because it's enjoyable, and that supports the belief that the work was fun—and thus potentially less stressful.

This quiz, adapted from one by researcher Teresa Amabile, will help you determine whether you lean more toward internal or external motivators. *Answer yes or no to the following statements:*

When you're faced with a difficult problem, is your
     response "Bring it on, baby"?
Do you prefer to figure out challenges at work by
     yourself?
Even if you fail at a new project, are you happy that you
     had a new experience?
Do you feel ambivalent about whether you get
     recognized for your accomplishments? Does work
     feel more like recess than work?
Are you able to offer up new ideas and not care what
     others might think of you?

Results: The more often you answer yes to these questions, the more likely it is that you're motivated by internal factors. And if not, maybe it's time for you to look for another job or at least revisit your motivation.

71. Optimize Your Work Environment

If you can make the office an empowering place, you can improve your health and decrease your stress. Some ways to do that:

Color: The U.S. Public Health Service did a two-year study of public buildings and found that when they analyzed the room with additional lighting and additional color there was a 5.5 percent production improvement. A combination of green and red seems to be the most productive. So-called ugly colors—white, black, brown—caused a drop in performance even on IQ tests by as much as twelve points in one study.

Light: Green light and blue light increase activity slightly, but a yellow light increases activity by about 30 percent.

Artwork and greenery: Keeping plants in the office gives us the feeling of living things, growing things; they're also healing, comforting, and empowering. Artwork can be edgy in lobbies to set a tone of innovation but shouldn't be edgy in the workplace because you want people to focus on the *work,* not on the artwork. Think natural and calming pieces.

Air quality: Sick-building syndrome has been reported by 23 percent of U.S. office workers, manifesting itself in such problems as respiratory ailments, allergies, and asthma. Push your bosses to make sure

the office has proper ventilation and clean air. Some
fragrances like lavender seem to help relieve stress,
and lemon reduces errors (bring your own lavender
and lemon aroma packs or sachets to work).

Temperature: Optimal productivity performance appears
to be at 72 degrees, and going too much colder is
associated with making more mistakes at work.

Humor: One of the secrets of a good office environment
is having people who can laugh and have fun. Now,
we're not saying you should be practicing your best
Chris Rock on your cube-mates (after all, everyone's
sensibilities are different), but maybe you should
embrace, not scorn, the office clown. He's just trying
to make you happier and healthier.

72. Control Your Workflow

While it would be a mistake for us to assume there's only
one way to work, we do think there are some traits and
behaviors that can make time and energy management a
whole lot easier. Some things you should consciously try
to integrate into your workday if you don't already:

❏ **Map your day:** Though you don't have to stick to an
exact schedule, you may get some stress relief if you
organize your tasks and not leave your day to total
chance. Don't work off the inbox . . . work off your
plan for the day. (Manage the inbox only after you've
done what you desire to do.)

❏ **Break often:** Take a walk for ten minutes every few

hours, have a bottle of water, clear your head. It's all part of energy management. The few minutes you spend away from your desk will make you more efficient when you get back.

❏ **Enlist troops:** We know that people are pretty stubborn when it comes to trying to accomplish goals on their own; they think it's a sign of failure if they show weakness or an inability to do a job. But you'll reduce stress (and save time) by asking for help when you need it. Don't be afraid to delegate or ask others to pitch in when you're overloaded (and offer to do the same for others when they're in tight spots).

❏ **Repurpose your lists:** Whether you work for a company or your family, we bet that you live and die by the list. Doesn't matter whether you use Post-its, a notebook, a wipe board, a PDA, or scraps of tissues—we want you to keep not only a to-do list but also an I-hate list. That is, when something bothers you in your job, write it down. Revisit the list in a week. If it's still bothering you, maybe it's time to aggressively pursue a solution (or another job). Our guess: Most of the time, those annoyances will be as fleeting as a one-hit wonder. And that should help you realize that it's the big picture, not the little one, that counts.

STRESS-MANAGEMENT TECHNIQUES:
FOR THE MIND AND SOUL

73. Learn from Buddhism

When some people think about meditation, the first association that pops into their minds is Buddhism. But most people know as much about Buddhism as they know about supernova nucleosynthesis. The goal of Buddhist meditation isn't to suppress emotions that are harmful (as many might expect) but rather to identify how they arise, how they are experienced, and how they influence us in the long run. For Buddhists, the good life isn't achieved by transcending an emotion—not even hatred—but by effectively managing it. The three mental processes that are most toxic to the mind (and that lead to all kinds of mental suffering) are:

❑ **Craving:** Me, mine, mmmm. Cravings happen when a person exaggerates the good qualities of an object (icing!) while ignoring the bad ones (calories!). Therefore, cravings can disrupt the balance of the mind, easily leading to anxiety, misery, fear, and anger.
❑ **Hatred:** The reverse of craving, hatred exaggerates the bad qualities and deemphasizes the good ones.

It's driven by the wish to harm or destroy anything that gets in your way. The impression is that the dissatisfaction belongs to the object, when the true source of it is in the mind alone.

❏ **Delusion:** According to Buddhism, the self is constantly in a state of dynamic flux and is profoundly interdependent with other people and the environment. However, people habitually delude themselves about the actual nature of the self by superimposing the interpretations of their own reality.

74. Think about Your Spirituality

Regardless of what motivates people to pray, there's no denying that a lot of people do it. One study shows that 36 percent of people use complementary and alternative medicine, but that number almost doubles when prayer is included in the definition. Those respondents say they use prayer for their own health and to help others. Even more telling: Of those people who said they prayed for health reasons, 70 percent said that prayer was helpful. Why? Seems as though it may work through several different mechanisms:

❏ **It relaxes:** A form of meditation (no matter what your religious preferences), prayer helps to slow breathing and brain activity, and reduces heart rate and blood pressure. All relaxing, all good.

❏ **It's positive:** Let's face it: When you pray, you typically don't finish feeling as though you want to rap somebody's ankles with a wooden spoon. Afterward you're filled with peace, joy, and other emotions that are worthy of being printed on holiday cocktail napkins. There's some evidence that these emotions lead to positive physiological responses throughout the entire body. Our stress hormone levels prepare for a peaceful existence.

❑ **It's better than nothing (i.e., the placebo effect):** We'd be remiss in our reporting if we didn't say that some of the benefits derived from prayer can be accounted for simply because the person feels as if it's helping, whether it's helping physiologically or not. (Placebo responses account for as much as 70 percent of the beneficial effect of some medical procedures and drugs. Our stance here is that thinking you're doing something to help yourself is a big part of prayer anyway.)

❑ **It's supernatural:** Perhaps the hardest reason to quantify, it's also one of the most powerful. Praying people believe in supernatural forces and in a god's ability to heal, and that seems to have a strong effect on their health—even if the real mechanism of effectiveness is through one of the three previous reasons. Now, no two mystics describe their otherworldly experiences in the same way, and it can be difficult to distinguish among the various types of mystical experiences, be they spiritual, traditionally religious, or simply awe-inspiring moments. If you're an atheist and you live a certain kind of experience, you will relate it to the magnificence of the universe. If you're a Christian, you'll associate it with God. The point, for us, isn't the differences between the spiritual experiences but rather the similarities—and that we can get to that place in lots of different ways.

75. Give, Then Pass

There are few feelings in the world that surpass knowing you've helped someone—whether it's through a financial donation or a mentoring program or giving up your seat on a crowded bus. It feels good—and is good. So good, in fact, that some researchers have found the effect of giving, of altruisms small and big, is similar to the so-called runner's high (the rush of endorphins). But unlike exercise euphoria, this rush can last a long time. The evidence: Ninety percent of people who experience this high give their health condition a better grade than those who don't. The reason: It seems that charity might really start at home. Your thoughts about helping others help you. They seem to be able to do things that strengthen your immune system, boost positive emotions, decrease pain, and provide stress relief. When you give something to somebody, we want you to find a way to allow them to have the dignity to pass it along to someone else. Though people very often need help, they also don't want to feel like charity cases. They want to feel that they can also pass something along to others. This also makes giving more attractive, since you are really priming the pump of a chain reaction that will help many more people than the one group you targeted with your kindness. So be explicit in your giving and ask how the recipient will pass it forward. Try to pick situations where this expectation is clear.

BONUS!
THE YOU STRESS
MANAGEMENT PLAN

Many of us have two thoughts about stress: Either you can eliminate it with a bubble bath, or you have to live with your stresses weighing on your mind with the weight of a cement truck. But the truth is, stress management isn't about eliminating it; after all, stress can be *good* for you. It's actually all about regulation—turning the dials of your emotions so you can best handle what life tosses at you. Stress, which is really a complex mix of emotional, physical, and behavioral responses, doesn't have to sideline you from life or send you straight to the ice-cream tub. Take a look at some more tricks to avoid letting your worries burden—or bury—you. And then use our 14-day plan (as well as deep-breathing and meditation guidelines) to help energize and revitalize you.

Stress Strategies
- ❑ Identify the source of your stress. Though some sources are easy to identify, it may be difficult to really determine what's bothering you. Lashing out

at your kids may be a reaction not to what your kids did but to an extra assignment piled on at work. The first step to managing your stress is pinpointing the culprit.

❑ **Focus on the moment.** Though it can be hard, you'll have better stress management by being "mindful"—that is, really paying attention to the present and trying to get out of the gears of the past and the future (both of which are major sources of stress). That means especially noticing the things that you ignore, like your breath, body sensations, and emotions. One way to practice living in the moment: the body scan. How do you do it? Focus on every part of your body, which will help you to relax:

❑ Lie down.

❑ Close your eyes and notice your posture.

❑ Think about the natural flow of your breath, focusing on air filling and leaving the lungs.

❑ Notice your toes—any tension, tingling, or temperature change?

❑ Move to thinking about your feet, heels, and ankles, all the way up through the knees, thighs, and pelvis.

❑ **Continue with each body part,** going through both the front and back of your body as you work your way up, and finishing with the throat, jaw, tongue, face, and brow.

❑ **Go through your health checklist:** Stress is much more manageable when the other aspects of your life—from your general health to your sleep patterns to your eating habits—are in good order. When you don't get enough sleep, for instance, your body produces more stress hormones, making you more vulnerable to the damaging effects of stress. Evaluate what areas in your life need your attention, and work on fixes.

❑ **Do the opposite:** Every emotion has an "urge to act" that goes with it. When we feel afraid or anxious, we avoid things; when we are depressed or sad, we withdraw (stay in bed). When we are angry, we want to lash out or yell. Unfortunately, each of these mood-inspired behaviors actually increases an emotion, not decreases it. However, if you can act the opposite way, you can decrease the emotion. Angry at someone? Don't lash out, but, rather, be empathetic. Depressed? Instead of shutting yourself in, go out. Rather than letting your emotions determine what you do, take control and choose how you feel.

❑ **Focus on your muscles:** By tensing and relaxing your muscles, you can help relieve some of your stored physical stress. While sitting or lying down, tense the muscles of your feet as much as you can and then release the tension. Tense and relax different muscle groups of your body one at a time. Focus on your legs, stomach, back, neck, arms, face, and head. When done, relax for a few minutes.

Deep Breathing and Meditation

Meditation and deep breathing may help modify the messages sent from the gut and the rest of the body to the brain via the vagus nerve. Controlling your vagus nerve can help you with everything from improving your memory to improving your immune system. We suggest you carve out time each day to breathe deeply and meditate. Before bed is a good time, or anytime when you're trying to manage stress.

❑ **Deep Breathing:** Lie flat on the floor, with one hand on your belly and one hand on your chest. Take a deep breath in slowly—it should take about five seconds for you to inhale (imagine your lungs filling up with air). As your diaphragm pulls your chest cavity down, your belly button should move away from your spine, filling your lungs. Your chest will also widen and perhaps rise. When your lungs feel full, and you even feel a tiny bit of discomfort in the solar plexus, just below the breastbone, exhale slowly (taking about seven seconds). Pull your belly button to your spine to get all the air out.

❑ **Meditation:** The goal here is to clear your mind of all thoughts. The first step: silence. Even if you use meditation only to sort out headache issues, discipline yourself to squirrel away five minutes of silence a day. To help clear your mind and meditate, pick a simple word (like ohm or Hawaii or supercalifrag—oh, you get the point) and repeat it to yourself over and over.

Focusing on the one word helps keep distracting thoughts from seeping into your gray matter.

The 14-Day De-Stress Plan

Day 1

Take a 30-minute walk.

Take 1 minute in a quiet room. Close your eyes and breathe deeply (see page 66). Focus on one word or image. If you are having trouble with this, try the "Stress Less" program from the www.clevelandclinic .org/wellness or www.360-5.com sites.

Give a compliment to someone who needs to hear one.

Make the Garden Harvest Soup (page 14) that you can keep on hand for the week to eat in case of hunger/ stress emergencies.

Day 2

Practice deep breathing for 2 minutes.

Try any 1 yoga move from our yoga workout.

Make plans to do something fun with a spouse, partner, friend, or relative on Day 6.

Day 3

Take a 30-minute walk.

Practice deep breathing for 2 minutes.

Substitute green tea for your usual "energy" drink.

Spend 2 minutes focusing on having good posture (see page 19).

Day 4

Practice deep breathing for 2 minutes.

For optimum energy and to avoid highs and lows, look
at your meals today and strive for balance between
protein, healthy fat, 100 percent whole-grain
carbohydrates. Make note of your energy levels
throughout the day.

Take a quick audit of your environment (work or
home) and see if you can identify things that
cause you stress. Purchase some lavender and
lemon aroma packs or sachets (you can find these
at aroma sections in health food stores or try
www.shopascents.com) to see if these help, and
brainstorm ways to eliminate (or reduce) that stress.

Day 5

Take a 30-minute walk.

Practice deep breathing for 3 minutes.

Write a thank-you note to someone unexpected about
something unexpected (and send it!).

Have the perfect late-afternoon snack instead of relying
on perhaps an energy crutch: We recommend a piece
of fruit and a handful of nuts.

Day 6

Practice deep breathing for 3 minutes.

Do the "something fun" you planned a few days ago.

Spend a few minutes and roll your neck in circles, then

rock it from front to back to help relieve tension
you're storing there.

Day 7

Take a 30-minute walk.

Practice deep breathing for 3 minutes.

Buy a pack of tennis balls. Take one and roll it over
chronically sore muscles, or places on your body
where you store tension.

Day 8

Practice deep breathing for 5 minutes.

Make a list of the nagging stresses in your life, then
brainstorm solutions for how to solve or eliminate
them.

Day 9

Take a 30-minute walk.

Practice deep breathing for 5 minutes.

Make a list of all the reasons why you love life; put it
somewhere where you'll take a look every so often.

Write a thank you note.

Day 10

Practice deep breathing for 5 minutes.

Make a smoothie that contains low-fat milk, non-fat
yogurt, a dab of natural peanut butter, ice, and your
favorite fruit—lots of nutrients, lots of energy.

Send an e-mail to an old friend you haven't talk to in
years (tell him or her you were thinking about them).

Day 11

Take a 30-minute walk.

Practice deep breathing for 5 minutes.

Try new yoga poses.

Day 12

Practice deep breathing for 5 minutes.

Add a plant to your office or other room where you
spend most of the day.

With your family or friends, make a "play" date—for
yourself. Choose a board game, a sport, something
that reminds you to get loose and have fun.

Day 13

Take a 30-minute walk.

Practice deep breathing for 5 minutes.

Try a few new yoga poses.

Day 14

Practice deep breathing for 10 minutes.

Swing on a swing, take a hike, go out and play.

Ask yourself the best way to help others. Make
arrangements to do just that.

APPENDIX

Look Great, Feel Great

You don't have to be a screen star to know that outer beauty matters. Simply, appearance is the proxy—the instant message to others—for youth, fertility, and health. And it's also a cycle that has a direct effect on stress. Looking your best can make you feel your best—and vice versa. In this bonus section, we'll show you the tricks that will help make your skin, hair, and teeth healthy, young, and beautiful. (More suggestions and science behind these at youbeauty.com.)

Your Skin: The Ideal Wash

Step 1. Watch What You're Washing

You have an acid mantle (like cellophane) that forms a protective layer on your skin to inhibit the growth of harmful bacteria and fungi. If it loses this acidity, the skin becomes more prone to damage and infection. How do you lose the acidity? By washing your face with ordinary soap. Most of the soaps we use are basic in nature, which counteracts the acidity, so you end up removing the mantle that seals in moisture. Now, we're not trying to encourage that outdoor look or manly smell by not washing. Use pH-balanced soaps and cleansers; if they are gentle enough not to sting your eyes, chances are good they won't harm your skin either. Your pores will look smaller if they're kept free of oils and dirt. Ideally, you should wash your face twice daily, and you don't need to spend more than a few seconds doing it. Excessive rubbing can aggravate eczema and acne. Skip the soaps with colors and fragrances, too. They just add residue and increase the chance of an allergic reaction.

Step 2. Add Anti-Oxis

If you read our tip on vitamins, you'll see how they can help improve the skin. Here's a quick recap of why polyphenols help: Natural polyphenols inside the membranes of your cells (vitamin E is the most common in the skin) protect you against free oxygen radicals in the membrane and lipid portions of the cell. They're especially important for protecting your skin, because they help thicken your epidermis while the sun quickly depletes levels of vitamin E. Your body will replenish its own vitamin E if you are eating smart, but adding some extra vitamin C (which protects the water-soluble portions of your cells) can help decrease the appearance of wrinkles and improve the formation of collagen and elastin. Only certain types of vitamin C will penetrate the skin—one called l-ascorbic acid does this particularly well. To work, it must be in a concentration of at least 10 percent and must be kept acidic. So, you can't just rub oranges on your face and expect it to work. l-ascorbic acid is oxidized by the sun, rendering it ineffective, so use it only at night. Topical application of niacinamide (niacin, vitamin B3) and pantothenic acid (vitamin B5) and other antioxidant vitamins (taken orally) are good for the skin. In fact, topical niacin helps prevent injury caused by the sun, and increases the level of certain fats and protein in the skin, which improves its barrier function, and it helps reduce the yellowing of skin that's associated with glycation (the yellowing can disappear after four to twelve weeks of use).

Step 3. Moisten Before Using

Typically, your skin soaks up moisture to keep itself young and vital, but it loses the ability to do that as you age. Most commercial face creams are oil-based and work by blocking the release of water from the skin. As people grow older, however, they cannot rely on oil-based preparations to block the release of moisture. That's because aged skin loses the ability to attract moisture in the first place and becomes fundamentally dehydrated. But the vitamin A family, commonly called retinoids, can increase the actual water content of the skin without clogging the dead layer of cells. Retin-A contains retinoic acid and requires a prescription. Retinyl propionate, retinyl palmitate, and retinol (retinaldehyde) don't require a prescription, and all are converted by your skin's own enzymes into retinoic acid. Healthy moisturizers don't disturb the acid mantle of the skin or clog pores. We prefer natural moisturizers, such as squalene (made from olives), avocado oil, walnut butter, or cocoa butter, and ones that are proven to be hypoallergenic. Apply while you're still damp from the shower to seal the moisture in, and remember, it's especially important to moisturize when you're flying, at high altitudes, or in dry climates.

Step 4. Exfoliate Often

Which is better for your floor? Sweeping it clean every week or waiting for all the gunk to build up and then doing one big power wash a year? Exactly. You have several choices when deciding to do the same with your face:

- ❑ Mop it clean daily or weekly with a light physical exfoliant or a chemical exfoliant. Don't use physical exfoliants that have sharp edges, since they can damage healthy skin below. Apricot seeds are natural and work like an old-fashioned straw broom as opposed to the newfangled chemical beads, which are more symmetrical like a synthetic broom. We favor the latter but won't report you to the authorities if you insist on going the old-fashioned way. Try some on the back of your hand to make sure it's not too harsh.
- ❑ Microdermabrasion is industrial-level exfoliation and can be repeated monthly for the best results in people with typical skin. Microdermabrasion uses either aluminum oxide or salt crystals or, even better, embedded diamonds to exfoliate while the oils are

sucked right out of those pores. See below for more about microdermabrasion.

- ❏ Power wash it with something stronger, like trichloroacetic acid, which takes off the top layer of skin (it looks so bad for a week that we recommend doing this once yearly around Halloween). This is most useful to lessen that annoying splotchy brown pigmentation. This requires a doc.
- ❏ Every few years you can scrape it with a sandblaster or wire brush—that's real dermabrasion and the recovery is not particularly pleasant, so new light lasers are being developed to do this without the downtime. Unfortunately, they're so new we can't recommend one yet.

While they all can be effective, it makes the most sense to us to exfoliate once a week to remove dead skin cells and stimulate growth of new ones. If you wear makeup or are exposed to a lot of dirt, exfoliating nightly is recommended (don't do it at midday, which basically only removes your makeup). Also, for the women here, you produce more oil during your period, so you're susceptible to more acne, meaning you should use a lighter peel. Use a loofah sponge for your body. The loofah mechanically removes the old layer of skin. (Turkish baths require loofahs, and folks don't feel really clean unless they've had a vigorous rubdown.) If you're going to do it yourself, look for exfoliating products that contain acids compatible with your skin's own natural acidity. Some options:

❑ Alpha hydroxy acid (usually listed as glycolic acid) works as an exfoliant by peeling off the top layer of dead skin and hydrating with moisturizer. Alpha hydroxy acids (skin-rejuvenating fruit acids) have been around for about twenty years and make a marked improvement in skin quality by sloughing dead skin cells off the surface so that more youthful-appearing fresh cells become visible. Fine lines and wrinkles lessen, and your skin takes on a fresher-looking tone.

❑ Glycolic acid (less than 10 percent concentration is safest; docs use higher concentrations), which is derived from sugarcane, traps moisture in skin and releases dead cells. Use it sparingly at first to make sure it doesn't cause skin irritation.

❑ Hyaluronic acid is a large sugar-like molecule in the extracellular matrix that binds with water and provides volume and fullness for skin, making skin smooth and moist. Hyaluronic acid can't penetrate the skin, however, so when you put it on your skin, it's really just a moisturizer.

❑ Apple cider vinegar also works as an exfoliant for the top layer of skin.

Step 5. Pick the Block

You're supposed to get twenty minutes of sunlight a day—but only when it's at low levels (a good rule of thumb: Your shadow should be longer than your height). This rule applies even on a cloudy day, which stops only

20 to 40 percent of UV radiation. Beyond that, you know the drill. You know it, you hear it, you see the ads with the baby's butt on billboards. Wear sunscreen. Like punishment doled out in the principal's office, sun protection is nonnegotiable—because it's the most critical factor in keeping skin healthy. It's best to make sunscreen a part of your daily regimen so you won't get unexpected exposure (or get a sunburn). Use a great moisturizer that you love that also contains an SPF 30 sunscreen and affords the protection you need. If you're going to be outside for sports, use a lotion with SPF 30 (for UVB) and a four-star rating (for UVA) and reapply every two hours. Our recommendation: Always protect your face and the backs of your hands but allow your body to be exposed to some sun for a few minutes before you add sunscreen. A little redness in the skin signifies that vitamin D is being made. Here's a helpful hint: Zinc oxide and titanium dioxide sunscreens protect immediately, and newer versions of these sunscreens form a thin film rather than making you look as if you smeared crayon all over your face. (We prefer zinc oxide, as titanium dioxide takes on an ashen color when mixed with certain sweat ingredients.) All the rest of the sunscreens—called chemical or organic sunscreens (misnomers if we ever heard one)—take twenty minutes to absorb into your skin before protecting. So get those few minutes of sun and then apply the zinc.

You need to slather all sunscreens on thickly and apply them evenly, making sure not to miss any spots such as the back of the neck, the top of the ears, and any exposed scalp. Most of us don't put on enough sunscreen, and if that's the case with you, then you're getting only half the effectiveness (if you're putting on SPF 30, it's more like SPF 15). You really need 1–2 ounces of sunscreen to cover your whole body. That's a Ping-Pong ball's worth for just face, neck, arms, and hands for the typical person. Which product is the best? Look for ones that are hypoallergenic and noncomedogenic, because you don't want to cause other skin damage while trying to protect from sun damage. But don't put a lot of faith in those labels, since all creams can cause pimples and rashes. It's really hit or miss. Also make sure that your sunscreen is water-resistant, so it doesn't end up in your eyes while the rest of the players on your team watch you drop the ball in painful anguish. Water-resistant also means it will stay on your body past the first droplet of sweat when you are hot. But even if it says "water-resistant," reapply it after swimming. By the way, hats and T-shirts don't provide enough SPF protection. Hats provide an SPF of 10 at the most, and T-shirts only about SPF 5 (but sun-protective clothing with higher SPFs are available). And wear sunglasses that filter the sun's UV rays to protect your eyes. Ever wonder what the heck the SPF numbers truly mean? An SPF of 1 means that your skin covered in SPF 1 would turn red in about twenty minutes; SPF 2 would require forty minutes, and so on. The most common reason for sunscreen failure is using inadequate amounts.

Step 6. Have a Pro Save Your Face

While some cosmetic procedures may seem as unnecessary as gumball machines, there are a lot of advantages to getting regular facials or microdermabrasion. Microdermabrasion is really a facial without all the glitz. It simply exfoliates your skin and sucks the dirt out of your pores. If you can afford it, get a facial or microdermabrasion monthly to clear pores, which can be clogged by makeup. The massage part will also stimulate blood flow. These cleaning procedures must be followed by proper skin care at home twice a day—cleaning, antioxidant protection, hydrating, protecting against the sun, and exfoliating regularly.

Your Hair: Perfect Maintenance
(see more at youbeauty.com)

Step 1. Shampoo

Before getting into the shower, gently brush or finger-comb your hair to loosen up tangles and residue. When washing your hair, treat it as if it were fine silk—delicately. Leave hair hanging down and gently massage in shampoo starting at the roots and working down. Never pile shampoo on top of your head.

Step 2. Condition

Conditioner creates shine and preserves hair health by giving it smoothness and protecting against damage. For volume, condition only the middle and ends of your hair, where it's most susceptible to damage. For shine, condition the entire strand. Do it every time you use shampoo and more often if you want.

Step 3. Dry

Don't rub your hair with a towel or twist it tightly into a turban. Wet hair is delicate and breaks easily. Pat it gently and squeeze it with your towel, or use a superabsorbent towel sold at salons. A wide-toothed comb is the best way to detangle and distribute styling products when hair is wet. And keep any dryers at low-heat settings.

Step 4. Practice Good Hair Hygiene

Most of what we do to hair is hairicidal: We blast it with hot air, bleach it, and then dye it. High hair-dryer heat (and that from curling irons) causes the water under the cuticles (the outermost layer of the hair) to form bubbles that stress and break the hair. The tiles that cover the hair dislodge, and your hair handles water like an unroofed house. You'll get those dreaded split ends, and your collie's hair will outshine yours. It's best to blot hair dry with a towel and then use low heat if you use a dryer. Your hair is actually most vulnerable when it's wet, and you should treat your hair almost as you would a silk blouse—don't iron it or heat it up to extremes. Also, it's smart to use a brush with smooth or rounded teeth or bristles, which will massage the hair and scalp without damaging them. Still, we also know that changing hair color can be an appearance advantage if it makes you feel better and healthier. And you know that we're going to quote Billy Joel when it comes to bleaching, dying, and adding hot-pink high-lights: We like you just the way you are.

Your Teeth

Waiting in traffic, two minutes seems like an eternity. Playing in bed, two minutes feels like a flash. At the sink, two minutes is the time you need to spend brushing your teeth to clean them adequately and reduce plaque. Use a soft brush and rub the bristles up toward the gums, so you can get to the actual cusps and gum. Change your toothbrush every two months. Those newfangled ultrasonic brushes amaze many dentists with their plaque-fighting abilities (and some have two-minute timers built in). Many cultures, by the way, believe that massaging your gums with your fingers is helpful in preventing periodontal disease. We actually prefer sonic brushes, since they produce more than thirty thousand brushstrokes a minute (compared to about five thousand of typical electrical ones) and spray into the crevices of teeth to clean beyond where the tips of the bristles actually touch. In other words, they're more effective at dislodging plaque. To use one, follow these instructions:

- ❑ Wet the bristles and use a small bit of toothpaste.
- ❑ Place the toothbrush bristles against the teeth at a slight angle toward the gum line. Power up.
- ❑ Apply light pressure to let the brush do the brushing for you (as with a sensitive coworker, don't push too hard).

❏ Gently brush the head slowly across the teeth in small back-and-forth motions so the longer bristles reach between your teeth.

❏ Do the outside top teeth, inside top teeth, outside bottom teeth, and inside bottom teeth each for thirty seconds. Then do the chewing surfaces and anywhere else that may have stains. Feel free to brush your tongue, too, which can help with bad breath.

❏ Floss for two minutes as well.